To Kirsty.
Love from
Mum xx

GW00722745

Good Housekeeping

salon
facials
at home

Rosie Mills

series editor
Vicci Bentley

HarperCollins*Illustrated*

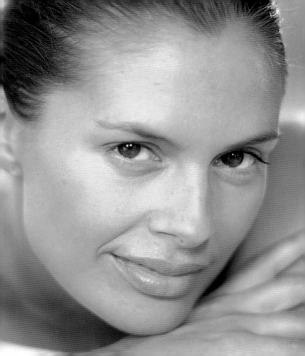

contents

Treating yourself to a regular facial is a blissfully relaxing and uplifting experience. It is also one of the best beauty investments you can make for achieving – and maintaining – a supple, fresh and healthy-looking complexion.

Today, salon facials are a popular and important part of any good skin-care regime. Beauty salons include at least one kind of facial or another in their treatment programme.

introducing facials

As a deep-cleansing, exfoliating and nourishing intensive treatment, facials are designed to do much more than just purify and refresh. Using special massage techniques, they also ease muscle tension, improve skin elasticity, circulation and lymphatic draining, diminishing dark circles around the eyes and help to reduce bags and puffiness. Though a facial will not banish wrinkles, like a surgical face-lift, frequent facials will work like a natural face-lift, brightening, tightening and firming up your skin to make those fine expression lines and wrinkles look much less marked.

So how do you achieve glowing, polished-smooth skin when you don't have the hours – or money – to spend at a beauty salon? *Salon Facials at Home* is your in-depth guide to an easily achievable, salon-professional facial. With effective, inexpensive and fun home-treatments that marry ease with results, you will soon start to realise why beauty experts regard a good facial not as a luxury but a necessity.

nothing beats massage
when it comes to
creating a bright,
supple complexion.
Your skin will
look fresher and
younger.

facial

massage

your
hands
are highly sensitive.
Using different parts
of them in
massage
will stimulate and
nourish skin.

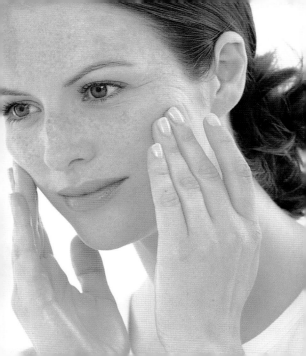

Effleurage, or skimming over: stroking your face can calm and relieve a tired and stressed mind and body. Apply light pressure to the area you want to work on. With moving hands, allow one hand to follow the other, in a rhythmic pattern.

Finger ball: use the balls of your fingers to stimulate nerve endings and galvanise blood vessels and lymph glands into action. Apply small circular

massage moves

movements to the relevant areas, press to a depth that feels comfortable.

Palming: the palms of your hands have a powerful, healing action with lots of nerve junctions that radiate heat. To help lymphatic drainage and guard against toxic build-up, repeat a simple stroking action using the palms for several minutes.

Pinching or kneading: fast-acting pinching will activate the nerve endings in your skin

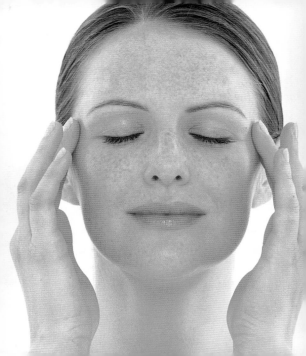

Use your thumb and index finger to pinch small areas like your forehead.

When massaging use a fine oil like almond or jojoba to avoid dragging the skin. Alternatively, add 3 drops of essential oil that is suited to your skin type with 1 tbs of carrier oil.

Caution: do not massage any sore or broken skin areas.

Facial tension can leave your complexion looking tired and lifeless. Pressing on the following acupressure points will release locked muscles, relieve congested areas and revitalise both your face and expression to help prevent premature ageing.

Treat each pressure point by applying a deep pressure with fingertips, then releasing it. Carry out this 'pumping action' 60 times, for about one minute. To relieve a headache and a hangover: touch your forehead, then press in a line from the centre of the hairline to the crown of your head.

friendly pressure

To relieve migraines and headaches try one or all of the following: touch the small indentation in the middle of the top of the eyebrow, then press • touch the top edge of your cheekbone directly below the pupil of your eye looking straight ahead, then press • press between your eyebrows • press below the end of each eyebrow.

To relieve sinus and tired eyes: press on the inside corner of your eyes.

To relieve sinus, facial tension or to clear nasal congestion: press on the small groove at the side of nose.

devoting five minutes in the morning and evening to facial massage will disperse bags and puffiness.

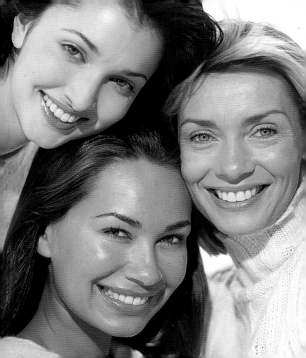

one Put your hands over your face and draw hands out towards your ears.

two Tilt your head to the left. Using the back of your hands, firmly stroke up the right side of your neck from your collar bone to your chin, one hand following the other. Repeat on the other side.

three Starting under your chin and working out to your ears, pinch all along the jaw-line using your thumbs and the knuckles of your index fingers.

four With alternate hands, slap under your chin with the backs of your hands.

five Using both hands, make small,

20

the DIY facial massage

circular pressure movements with your index and middle fingers. Massage over your chin and around your mouth.

six With one hand on each cheek, move them both out together, stroking from the corners of your mouth, out to your ears.

seven With one hand following the other, stroke up to your forehead from the bridge of your nose to your hairline.

eight Massage the muscle between your eyebrows making short, firm strokes. Stroke upwards first, then across and, finally, diagonally.

nine Make circular pressure movements all over your forehead, followed by gentle stroking with your fingertips. Work from the centre out to the temples. Finish by pressing gently on the temples. **ten** With your middle fingers, gently stroke in a circle around your eyes, from the bridge of your nose and then out over your eyebrows. Press on your temples, then glide lightly under the eyes. **eleven** With your thumbs and index fingers, pinch along your eyebrows from the centre to the temples.

twelve Refresh eyes by palming –
place the heel of your hands into your
eye-sockets. Press gently. Slowly glide
hands away. Finish by covering your
face with your hands and stroking
gently out sideways.

Tip: energise your skin with brisk,
fast massage actions. Soothe and
unwind with slow, calming
movements. As tension in your neck is
reflected in your face, massage over
your neck area too.

For tired, puffy eyes

1 tbs egg white • 1 tsp ground almonds •
1 small sprig fresh rosemary • 100 ml (3 fl oz)
boiling water

Put the sprig of rosemary in a bowl and pour on
boiling water. Cover and leave to cool, then
remove rosemary sprig and strain. Next, put the
ground almonds in a bowl and mix in the egg
white and 2 tbs of the rosemary infusion. Gently
dab the mixture under your eyes. Lie down and
relax for 15 minutes. Rinse off with warm water
and pat dry. Egg white can be drying so lightly
massage the area with almond oil.

24

facial trouble-shooting

For frown lines

50 ml (2 fl oz) rose water • contents of 1 vitamin E capsule • 2 drops frankincense oil • 50 g (2 oz) ground almonds • cotton pads

Put the rose water in a bowl. Add the oil. Stir in the ground almonds and vitamin E to make a paste. Smooth ½ tsp of the paste over the centre of a cotton pad. Lay the pad, paste-side down, over frown lines. Relax for 45 minutes. Remove and rinse off. Apply moisturiser.

For a slack jaw-line or a double chin

Rub a small amount of almond oil into your hands. In a sweeping action, gently stimulate the jaw-line from the centre of your chin and out to your ears, using the palms of your hands. Repeat night and morning.

26

For dark circles under the eyes

Grate a small potato or cucumber. Divide into two. Place each portion between two small squares of muslin, cheesecloth or an old clean handkerchief. Use squares as under-eye packs. Leave pads on the eyes for 20 minutes.

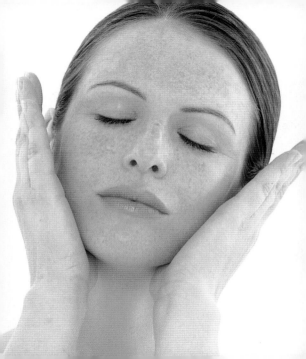

deep-cleansing is fundamental to a healthy, youthful-looking skin. To achieve fresh, glowing skin that doesn't age rapidly you need to get the basics right.

deep

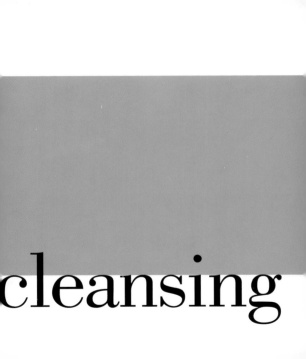

cleansing

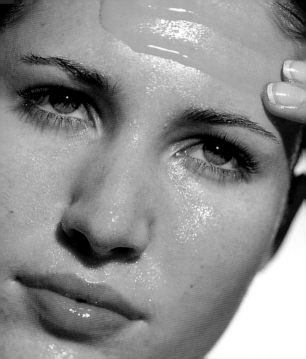

deep-cleansing systems have the power to improve the condition of your skin, keeping it healthy and spot-free.

For healthy skin you need to take regular exercise, eat a balanced diet and practise an effective skin-care regime that starts with deep-cleansing. At the end of the day, your skin can suffer from a build-up of sebum, sweat and dead-skin cells that can make your complexion uncomfortably greasy and sticky. Airborne dust, pollens and particles from vehicle-exhaust fumes, particularly if you live in a city, can also

coming clean on skin

become ingrained in your skin's epidermis – its outermost layer. Dirt can block hair follicles, encouraging pimples and make your skin look less than its best. Add to this a day of wearing make-up and you can see why it is essential to cleanse your skin daily, and also to deep-clean your skin on a regular basis. For your facial-intensive, couple ultra deep-cleansing with a deep-clean steam.

don't forget
your neck
– think of your
face as the zones
from your collar
bones to
your hairline.

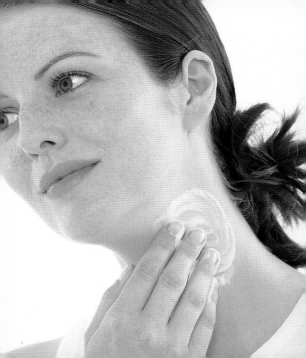

To deep-cleanse go gently but thoroughly, applying a light layer of cleanser to your face, lips and neck. Leave for a few minutes to allow make-up and dirt to dissolve. Using a damp cotton-wool pad, wipe away grime and cellular debris by working upwards from the neck in firm sweeping movements. When the cotton pad is clean, you are finished. Rinse your face and neck with water or apply a gentle toner. If you are using an eye make-up remover, go gently, make sure that you do not tug or pull at the delicate skin around the eyes.

gently but thoroughly

Many professional facials start with steaming to soften the skin, open the pores and release hidden dirt and debris. To deep-clean with steam, hold your face about 30 cm (12 in) above a bowl of boiling water, covering your head with a towel. Steam for 5 minutes if your skin is dry, increase this to 10 minutes if your skin is oily. Do not steam too frequently as delicate facial skin is exposed to an unusual heat during this treatment. For normal, or oily skin, once a week is fine. For dry skin, every two weeks is sufficient.

For a fragrant facial steam, add a few drops of essential oil, or try all-skin-type herbs such as chamomile, elderflower, comfrey, nettle or linden flower.

38 Caution: do not steam-clean your face if you have sensitive skin, broken skin or broken veins.

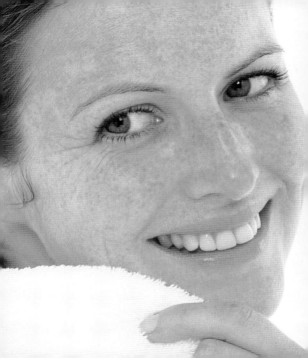

Each morning, do a simple wipe-over with a dampened cosmetic pad to remove surface oil and dead skin-cells after the night-time repair work to skin has taken place. Every evening, thoroughly remove the day's grime and make-up. For your

deep-cleansing facial, make sure you are using the appropriate cleanser for your skin type.

For dry, delicate or mature skin use a cream cleanser that has a rich consistency and leaves a light, moisturising film.

- For normal-to-oily and oily skin use a foaming or gel cleanser to help dissolve any oil-based residue and make-up.
- For normal and normal-to-dry skin use a lotion with a combination of mild detergents and moisturisers so they do not strip the skin of vital oils.
- For acne-prone skin use a gentle gel or foaming cleanser – but do go easy on the scrubbing.
- For sensitive, allergy-prone skin use a lotion or cream that is free from possible allergens and well-known irritants such as lanolin and perfume.

For combination skin it may be necessary to use two products – one for the greasy area, another for the drier parts.

Caution: soap isn't that efficient at dissolving make-up and can strip natural oils from the skin. Opt for a soap-free facial cleansing bar instead.

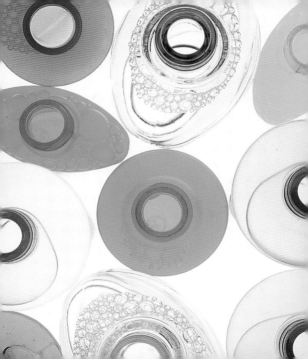

gently assisting the
departure of dead
surface-skin cells which
might otherwise clog pores
will refine skin
texture to leave it clear,
smooth and
translucent.

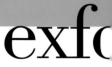

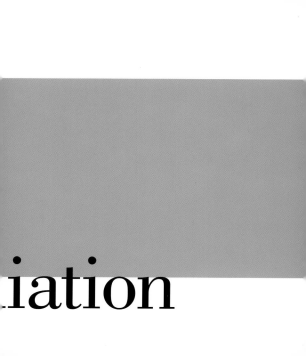

iation

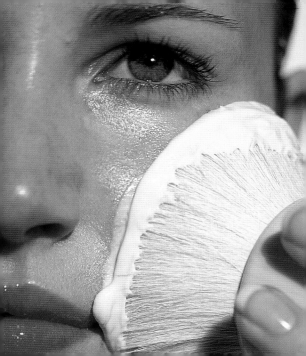

the key to
fresher
looking skin
is exfoliation,
make sure
to include it in
your weekly
routine.

After the age of about 25 cell turnover diminishes gradually and skin can appear dull, tired and grey. To help speed up the renewal process and improve blood circulation, exfoliate. Exfoliation – a mild form of peeling – is an essential part of your DIY facial. As your skin grows new cells, it casts off the old. Sloughing off these dead, flaking cells will not only stimulate cell regeneration, it will also banish rough skin, stop

why exfoliate?

spots and blackheads appearing, and allow your skin to reflect light more effectively. The gentle massaging involved in exfoliation brings the added benefit of flushing your skin with fresh blood and oxygen. Another good reason to exfoliate is to prepare your skin for the moisture-powered lotions and facial masks you have selected for your facial, allowing them to penetrate through to the new layer of skin both faster and more effectively. Exfoliate gently after cleansing, followed by a moisturising cream or mask. Repeat two or three times a week.

50 Caution: sun-lovers take note. Newly exfoliated skin is more vulnerable to sun damage. If you are going out in the sun, remember that you need to apply a sun block.

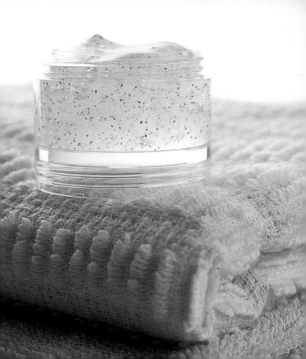

The simplest form of exfoliation is to rub your face with water and a coarse-textured sponge. You can also exfoliate dead cells by rubbing gently with a face cloth or towel. For your home-facial, a more effective skin sloughing treatment should involve a home-made scrub, applied to damp skin, using a natural exfoliate such as oatmeal which is perfect for all skin types including sensitive and acne-prone skin. Use

when and how often?

your finger tips to buff away dull surface cells from your forehead, cheeks and chin using small, circular movements. Wipe your neck, nose and the perimeters of your face in a vertical motion. Try to concentrate on the oily parts, avoiding the area around your eyes. Finally, rinse your face and neck with tepid water and gently pat dry. As you age exfoliation is a vital part of your skin-care regime.

A gentle facial scrub for all skin types

2 heaped tsp fine oatmeal • 2 tsp double cream
Combine both ingredients, and apply to your face
and neck with a very light massage action using
the balls of your fingers. Rinse off and moisturise.

54 A mild facial scrub for normal, dry and mature
skin

2 tsp honey • 2 tbs ground almonds • 4 tbs
natural yoghurt • 2 drops rose oil (optional)
Combine the honey and ground almonds in a
bowl. Add the yoghurt to make a thick paste. Beat
in the rose oil. Apply, avoiding the area directly
around your eyes. Gently massage the mixture

what to use?

onto your face and neck. Leave for two minutes, then rinse off, and moisturise.

The five-minute facial scrub for oily skin

2 tbs natural yoghurt • I tsp lemon juice
• 2 tbs cornmeal

Put the cornmeal in a bowl and add the lemon juice and yoghurt. Mix to make a paste. Leave for five minutes while the cornmeal softens. Gently massage the paste over your face, avoiding the area around your eyes, for five minutes. Rinse off and pat dry, then moisturise.

For a soft, smooth complexion, try this gentle recipe that is particularly good for dry and sensitive skin.

2 tbs natural yoghurt • 2 tbs fine oatmeal • I tbs almond oil (omit if you suffer from acne)

Put the oatmeal in a bowl and gradually add the almond oil and yoghurt. Mix and leave the oatmeal to soften for five minutes. Gently massage the mixture over your face and neck, avoiding the area around your eyes. Relax for five minutes. Rinse off with tepid water and pat dry. Then tone and moisturise.

First cleanse your skin. Wrap a face cloth around your index finger and lubricate it with a facial cleansing soap. Make small circular movements over your nose, twice. Rinse off and apply your facial scrub, using the same small circular actions over your nose to dislodge any debris or blackheads.

57

Cleanse, buff and polish the surface of your skin morning and night to maintain a fresh, smooth, glowing complexion.

A cleansing regime for dry skin

step one: to cleanse

am: a gentle wipe with a damp cotton pad

pm: apply a rich cream cleanser

step two: to exfoliate

am: a gentle rub with towel or face cloth

pm: a dry-skin scrub.

cleansing regimes

A cleansing regime for oily skin

step one: to cleanse

am: a thorough wipe with a damp cotton pad

pm: wash with a foaming or gel cleanser

step two: to exfoliate

am: a gentle rub with a towel or face cloth

pm: an oily-skin, five-minute facial scrub.

A cleansing regime for combination skin

step one: to cleanse

am: a gentle wipe – more thoroughly over oily patches – with a damp cotton pad

pm: a foam or gel cleanser over oily patches. Lotion or cream over the rest of your face.

step two: to exfoliate

am: a gentle rub with a towel or face cloth

pm: an oily-skin, five-minute facial scrub on greasy areas. A gentle facial scrub over the rest of your face.

A cleansing regime for sensitive skin

step one: to cleanse

am: a gentle wipe with a damp cotton pad

pm: an irritant-free lotion or cream

step two: to exfoliate

am: a gentle rub with a towel or face cloth

pm: a gentle facial scrub or dry-skin scrub.

A cleansing regime for mature skin

step one: to cleanse

am: a gentle wipe with a damp cotton pad

pm: a rich cream cleanser

step two: to exfoliate

am: a gentle rub with a towel or face cloth

pm: a mild facial scrub.

Caution: scrubbing too hard can cause
broken veins.

mix up your own glorious cocktail of active natural ingredients, tailored to suit your skin type. A facial mask can help rebalance many mild skin problems.

facial

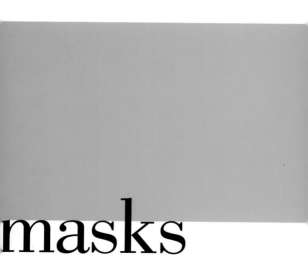

masks

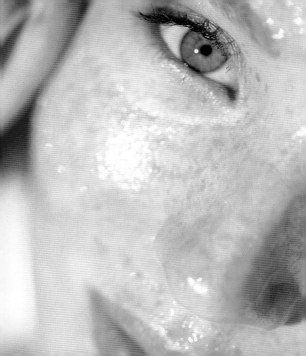

giving yourself a once-a-week facial mask will not only benefit your skin, it will also provide you with a restful break.

Masks leave your skin feeling fresh and smooth. Depending on the ingredients, they deep-cleanse, exfoliate, stimulate circulation or generally refine your complexion. You don't need to splash out on expensive masks as you will have most of the ingredients you will need at home. Fresh fruit and vegetable masks are a boon for sensitive skins because they contain no chemical preservatives. For dry skin try melon,

home-made masks

avocado, egg yolk, cream, honey, and banana. To tighten oily skin try beaten egg white, yoghurt, lemon, oatmeal, cucumber, parsley, ground almonds and yeast. Honey is valued for its soothing and mildly antiseptic qualities (use the runny variety). Lemon juice is known for its cleansing and anti-bacterial properties. Double cream is a natural skin food containing vitamins A, D and E.

Normal skin needs a hydrating, rejuvenating or firming facial mask to promote radiance.

Combination or oily skin needs a stimulating mask with a purifying, exfoliating action. You may need to use two types: one for the oily areas and another for the drier parts.

Dry skin needs a calming or hydrating mask with nourishing and moisturising ingredients such as honey, cucumber and banana.

masks for all skin-types

- Mature skin, dry and sensitive skin needs a nourishing creamy mask to rejuvenate and hydrate the skin. Use ingredients such as honey and yoghurt that won't set hard.
- Irritated and sensitive skin needs a calming mask that contains soothing ingredients such as cucumber.
- Dull, lifeless and tired looking skin needs a rejuvenating or stimulating mask that exfoliates the skin to remove dead cells and stimulate cell renewal.

Lightly apply the facial mask to cleansed skin, avoiding the area around your eyes and mouth. On your neck, work upwards from the base, smoothing on the mask evenly and right up to the edges of your face. Leave on for the specified time. Rinse off with water, pat skin dry and moisturise.

A calming facial mask

1 tbs softened unsalted butter

• Dry skin: 1 egg yolk.

• Normal to oily skin: 1 large strawberry mashed

• Normal to dry skin: a 2.5 cm (1 in) slice of cucumber, chopped and rubbed through a sieve.

specific action recipes

• Normal to oily skin: 1 tbs lemon juice

In a bowl, beat the butter then add your selected ingredients. Smooth onto your face and rest for 15 minutes. Rinse off and pat dry.

A hydrating facial mask

½ banana • 2 tbs natural yoghurt • 1 tbs honey

Mash the banana and add the honey and yoghurt. Mix to a smooth paste. Smooth over skin and rest for 10–20 minutes. Wash off and pat dry.

Caution: remove immediately should you feel any discomfort.

A stimulating facial mask

2 tbs chopped parsley (good for oily skin)
• 3 tbs fine oatmeal • juice of ½ large grapefruit
Put the oatmeal and parsley in a bowl. Gradually
mix in the grapefruit juice – just enough to
make a loose paste which will spread. Soften for
5 minutes and then apply evenly over your face.
Rest for 15 minutes. Rinse off and pat dry.

A rejuvenating facial mask

1 egg • 1 tbs sunflower oil • 1 drop lavender oil
Blend the egg and cooking oil and then add the
lavender. Apply evening and rest for 15 minutes.
Rinse off and pat dry.

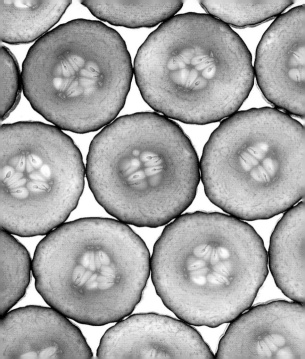

The first facial zone to reveal your age is the eye area. Smooth on a softening eye mask when skin looks tired and use fresh natural-ingredient refreshers. Always wait at least half an hour before applying your eye make-up.

74 Mask to refresh puffy eyes

Cut a fig in half and lie down for 10 minutes with fig pads on your eyes. Or, put 1 or 2 tsp of grated potato onto 2 squares of tissue paper (big enough to cover eyelids) and place under eyes. Rest for 15–30 minutes. Remove and splash eyes with cold water.

eye masks

Mask to soften the lines around the eyes

1 tsp aloe vera gel • 1 tsp ground almonds
• 1 tsp herbal tea, made from an infusion of
1 tsp dried (2 heaped tsp chopped fresh) herb.

Normal skin: rosemary, chamomile, lime
flowers or nettle

Oily skin: lemon peel, sage, mint or
lavender flowers

Dry skin: parsley, borage or camomile

Cover the herbs with boiling water and steep
until cold. Strain. Mix ingredients together and
smooth onto skin above and below the eyes.
Rinse off with warm water.

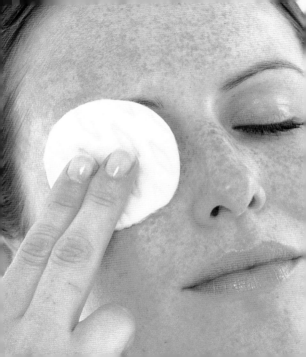

To banish the dark circles under your eyes and reduce puffiness

Soak two cotton-wool pads in cool-from-the fridge cornflower water. Place pads over lids. Rest for 15 minutes. Alternatively, try cold chamomile tea bags.

A quick fix for under-eye bagginess

Gently smooth on egg white under eyes to tighten skin. Leave to dry naturally before removing with water and wait for half an hour before applying your make-up.

therapeutic essential oils added to creams, lotions and oils will not only help soothe, refresh and rebalance your complexion, they will also have an effect on your mood.

arom

atherapy

The effectiveness of pure plant oils has been known for centuries. Extracted from all parts of a plant, these concentrated, uplifting essences will add a luxurious feeling to your DIY facial. They will also help hands to glide gently and easily over your face and neck while the oils are absorbed through the skin and into your blood stream. Many of the essential oils have antiseptic, anti-inflammatory and antibacter-

the benefits of plant oils

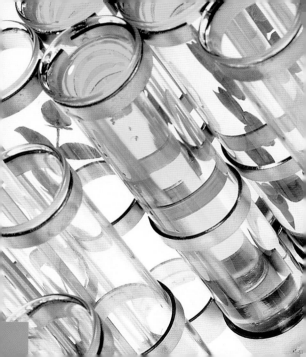

ial properties, coupled with many mood-enhancing benefits. Antiseptic ylang ylang can lift depression, restorative rose will energise, while astringent geranium can help dispel anxiety. As pure extracted oils, essential oils are highly concentrated and cannot be used directly on the skin. To avoid skin irritation, always dilute your essential oil first, either with a base lotion or in a base-carrier oil such as jojoba, grapeseed, apricot kernel, almond or pure wheatgerm oil (baby oil or cooking oil are not suitable). For facial massages, mix three to five drops of essential oil with one tablespoon of carrier oil or lotion, depending on how sensitive your skin is. Keep your aromatherapy facial oil in a plastic or glass bottle with a narrow opening so you can add a few drops of oil when massaging your face and neck.

Buy good-quality, pure essential oils and base oils from a reputable source. Store in a cool, dark place in air-tight bottles. Use within two years (one year in the case of citrus oils).

Bergamot: antiseptic and astringent. Excellent for acne and greasy skin. Do not use just before exposure to the sun.

Chamomile: skin-soothing. For sensitive and dry skin, rashes and thread veins.

Cedarwood: for oily skin.

Frankincense: antiseptic and soothing.

Geranium: uplifting and astringent. Tones the skin. Suitable all skin types.

oils for skin problems

Lavender: antiseptic, healing, soothing, relaxing and refreshing. Use undiluted.

Lemon: uplifting and refreshing.

Neroli (orange blossom): calming. Very good for dry skin and thread veins.

Petitgrain (leaves of the bitter orange): refreshing and particularly good for oily skin. A cheaper alternative to neroli.

Patchouli: calming and uplifting. Relieves stress and anxiety. An anti-inflammatory and antiseptic essential oil which is good for acne and eczema.

Rose: an expensive, restorative essential oil for dry and mature skins.

Sandalwood: suitable for dry dehydrated skin and can also be used as an antiseptic for acne.

Tea Tree Oil: antiseptic, soothing and healing. Good for the treatment of pimples and boils, no need to dilute.

Cypress: decongestant, astringent, revitalising oil, useful for hot flushes. Avoid during the first three months of pregnancy.

Eucalyptus: stimulating and antiseptic, eucalyptus oil is also highly decongestant.

Juniper: an antiseptic, healing revitalising oil, also a powerful detoxifier. Use in small quantities, don't use if pregnant.

Niaouli: a powerful antiseptic, anti-inflammatory, healing, regenerating oil. Helps relieve oily skin and acne.

Orange: a calming, anti-depressant oil, good as a skin tonic. Do not use before sun exposure.

Rosewood: less expensive and not as potent as rose oil. Good for dry skin.

Peppermint: antiseptic, energising. Use in small quantities and avoid in the first three months of pregnancy.

Mixing your own skin-care blend of fragrant essential oils is both intriguing and enjoyable. You will also know it's free from unwanted additives. If you want to add an essential oil to your moisturising facial cream or lotion put 2 drops of essential oil into 4 ml of a neutral lotion or cream base. Avoid the area around your eyes when applying.

Caution: at least an hour before applying a home-blended oil do a patch test, particularly if you have sensitive skin.

DIY blends

Dry-skin enricher

Add 24 ml of jojoba oil to 2 drops rose oil, 3 drops sandalwood oil, 4 drops neroli oil and 3 drops patchouli oil. Gently massage your face.

Freshener for all skin-types

120 ml (4 fl oz) still mineral water • 6 drops lavender oil

Put the lavender oil and mineral water into a sterilised, screw-top jar. Close container tightly and shake well. Transfer to a sterilised spray bottle. Splash or mist onto skin. Keep cool in the fridge and use within two weeks.

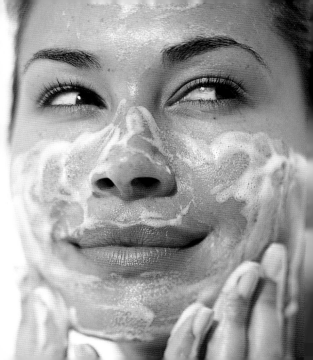

Anti-ageing compress for all skin types,
particularly mature skin

3 drops rose oil • 2 drops geranium oil • 1 tsp
avocado oil • 175 ml (6 fl oz) lukewarm mineral
water • Face cloth

Put the lukewarm water in a large, shallow bowl.
and add the oils. Place the face cloth over the
surface of water to absorb some of the oil.
Squeeze gently and place flannel over your
face, oily side down. Rest for 45 minutes, then
apply moisturiser.

Do dilute your highly concentrated essential oil first in a carrier oil to avoid skin irritation.

Do seek professional advice from a trained aromatherapist and/or doctor before using essential oils if you suffer from skin allergies, epilepsy, high blood pressure, are breast-feeding, pregnant, or have any other medical condition.

Do avoid directly inhaling pure essential oils if you are an asthmatic – they could bring on an asthma attack.

do's and don'ts

Don't take internally. Keep bottles out of reach of children. If swallowed, seek medical advice immediately.

Don't put near a naked flame.

Don't allow any essential oil to come into contact with plastic, polished or painted surfaces.

Don't let oils near your eyes. If affected, wash eyes immediately with plenty of water. Seek medical advice.

Don't expose skin to the sun after using oils as they accelerate the skin's reaction.

armed with your new
skin-care knowledge fo
creating the salon-perfect
facial at home, devise
your individual regime –
then get mixing for your
own DIY specials.

home

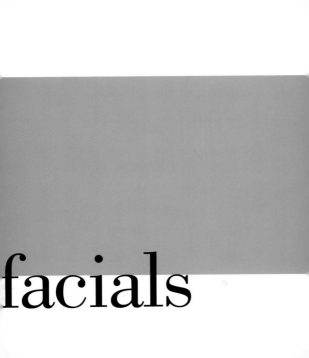

facials

Do not buy all the ingredients at once. Decide which ones you will be using for your immediate facial recipes and stock up accordingly. Make small quantities and keep any recipe containing perishable ingredients in the fridge.

Basic ingredients

Oatmeal • Almonds • Natural yoghurt • Pure essential oils • Carrier oil • Beeswax (optional) – prevents oils separating-out in creams and lotions • Cucumber • Potatoes • Eggs

facial checklist

Equipment

Cosmetic pads • Towels • Face cloth • Weighing scales • Measuring jug • Glass or china mixing bowls • Labels • Sterilised misting-spray bottle • Grater • Blender • Mortar and pestle • Wooden spoon • Tablespoons and teaspoons • Sharp knife and chopping board • Whisk • Double-boiler/bain-marie • Saucepan • Sterilised jars, pots and bottles with air-tight lids to store finished products.

Your basic skin type is down to genetics. It is also affected by changes in your diet, hormones, health and stress-levels. Exposure to sun, pollution, central heating and air conditioning can be tough on your complexion too. By focusing on how your skin's needs change, not only from season to season but from week to week, you can give your complexion the right treatment at the right time.

the six-step facial

Do not forget the golden skin rule: inner health means outer beauty. Drink two to three litres of water a day, enjoy plenty of sleep, stay out of the sun, and eat a low-salt, low-fat diet to keep skin looking radi- ant. Munching your way through five portions of antioxidant-containing fruit and vegetables each day will also help protect your skin from ageing as will exercise on a daily basis.

Massage cleanser over your face, lips and neck. Leave for a few minutes, then with a damp cosmetic pad, sweep upwards from neck until pad is clean. Steam-clean if you need to.

100

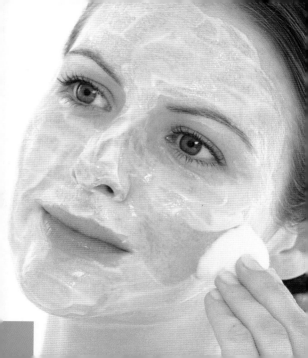

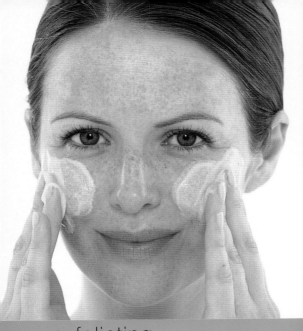

exfoliating

Tie back your hair. **Prepare your chosen scrub or mask. Using your fingertips, massage the mixture evenly over your face and neck, avoiding the area around the eyes. Wipe away and rinse off with** **tepid water.**

Using a fine base-carrier oil to avoid dragging skin, follow the technique described in DIY facial massage, or use one of the massage techniques to ease problem areas.

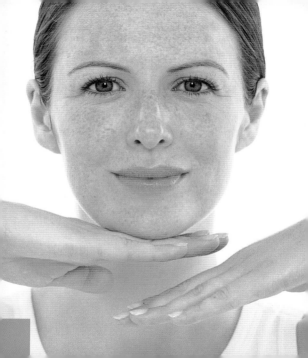

Gently and evenly apply your chosen facial mask avoiding the areas around your eyes and mouth. Apply mask to your neck also, working upwards from the base right up to the edges of your face.

facial mask

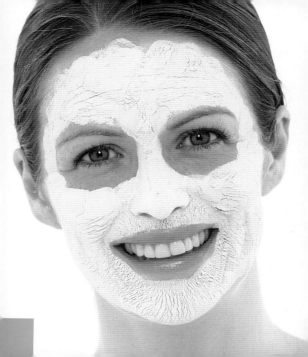

Cover a pillow with a towel. **Lie down, close your eyes and relax for the time your treatment takes. Breathe deeply and enjoy this extra special free-time.**

relaxing

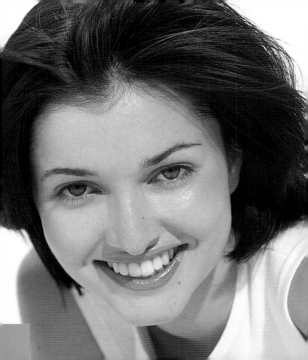

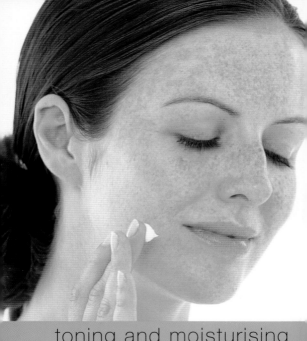

toning and moisturising

Gently remove the facial mask with a dampened cotton pad. Splash your face with one of the best toners of all – cold water. Pat dry and smooth on moisturiser while your skin is still damp.

First published in 2000 by
HarperCollins*Illustrated*
An imprint of HarperCollins*Publishers*
77–85 Fulham Palace Road
London W6 8JB

The HarperCollins website address is: www.**fire**and**water**.com

Published in association with The National Magazine Company Limited.
Good Housekeeping is a registered trademark of The National Magazine Company
Limited and the Hearst Corporation.

The Good Housekeeping website address is www.goodhousekeeping.co.uk

British Library Cataloguing-in-Publication Data
A catalogue record for this book is available from the British Library.
ISBN 0-00-710445-6

Colour reproduction by Colourscan, Singapore
Printed and bound in China by Imago